Top 50+ workouts For Seniors

(An Easy & Proven Way to Reclaim Balance, Strength, and Lose Weight)

By

Pilar Patel

Table Of Contents

Introduction

Imagine, just for a moment, me - Pilar Patel, stepping into the golden years, discovering something so powerful, so transformative, it felt like uncovering a secret garden in my own backyard. This was not just any discovery; it was the realization that even as the years add up, our bodies and minds are eager, almost pleading, for us to take control, to mold and improve through the art of exercise. This book, "Top 50+ Workouts for Seniors," was born from that very moment of enlightenment. It's not just a collection of exercises; it's a gateway to a new, invigorated phase of life, tailored specifically for us, the seasoned generation.

What sets this book apart? It's our unique blend of safety, specificity, and spirit. We delve into workouts that marry flexibility with strength, balance with endurance, all while ensuring the utmost safety—a critical aspect for us in our prime years. You'll find within these pages not just exercises, but stories of real-life transformations, easy-to-follow guides, and illustrations that bring clarity and motivation right to your fingertips.

Now, let me introduce myself properly. I'm Pilar Patel, a late bloomer in the fitness world, but a fervent believer in its power to rejuvenate and empower. My journey from a fitness novice to a passionate advocate for active aging is a testament to the fact that it's never too late to start. This book is my way of paying it forward, to help you, my fellow seniors, discover the joy and countless benefits of staying active.

Why is this so important? The evidence is clear. Physical activity is our ally against age-related decline, a beacon of hope for mental clarity, and a proven booster for our overall quality of life. By integrating regular exercise into our daily routine, we're not just moving our bodies; we're uplifting our spirits, sharpening our minds, and extending the quality of our years.

So, let's embark on this journey together, with an open heart and the will to embrace each day with vigor and zest. Remember, it's not about defying age; it's about redefining it. As I often say, "The best time to start was yesterday. The next best time is now." Let this book be your guide to a healthier, happier you. Together, we'll prove that age is but a number, and life, no matter the stage, is ripe for the taking.

Chapter 1:

The Unique Fitness Needs of Seniors

Embarking on a fitness journey at any stage of life is not just about movement; it's a declaration of defiance against the stereotypes and myths that often shackle the senior community. Let's shatter some of these myths together, shall we? The common misconception that seniors should reduce physical activity to avoid injury couldn't be further from the truth. Scientific evidence robustly supports the benefits of regular, moderate exercise for seniors, showcasing its role in enhancing mobility, reducing the risk of chronic diseases, and even improving mental health.

Safety, a valid concern, is often the shadow that looms over the decision to start exercising. However, the reality is that the risk of injury can be significantly minimized through tailored, senior-specific exercises that respect your body's limits and potential. Remember, countless seniors have embarked on their fitness journey later in life, proving that age is just a backdrop, not the protagonist of your story.

Exercise, in its magical essence, has the power to slow down certain aspects of the aging process, improving not just physical but mental well-being, enhancing cognitive function, and bolstering emotional resilience. It's about adding life to your years, infusing each day with quality and vitality.

Moving to the practicalities, assessing your fitness level is the foundational step in this journey. It's not about where you start but where you're willing to go. Begin with simple tests to gauge your current fitness level, setting the stage for realistic, achievable goals. These goals are your lighthouses, guiding you through the fog, keeping you motivated and on track.

However, remember, consulting with healthcare providers or fitness professionals before starting any new exercise regimen is crucial. They can offer invaluable insights into tailoring a program that aligns with your unique health profile and capabilities. Adaptation is key. Your fitness plan should be as unique as you are, designed not just for where you are now but where you dream to be.

In this chapter, we'll dive deep into these essential first steps, empowering you with the knowledge and confidence to start your fitness journey on the right foot. Together, we'll navigate through myths, set realistic goals, and craft a path that respects your individual needs and aspirations. It's a journey of transformation, not just of the body, but of the spirit and mind. Let's

The Unique Fitness Needs of Seniors: Safety Before, During, and After Workouts

Seniors embarking on a fitness journey have unique needs that must be carefully considered to ensure their safety and maximize the benefits of exercise. Recognizing these needs helps in creating a workout routine that is not only effective but also sustainable over time.

Here's a breakdown of what needs to be addressed for safety before, during, and after workouts:

I.   Before Workouts:

* **Medical Clearance:**
  Before starting any new exercise regimen, seniors should consult with a healthcare provider. This step is crucial for identifying any underlying health conditions that could affect their ability to exercise safely.

* **Personalized Fitness Plan:**
  Seniors should work with fitness professionals to develop a plan that considers their current fitness level, health conditions, and goals. This plan should include exercises that improve balance, flexibility, strength, and endurance, without putting undue strain on the body.

* **Proper Equipment and Environment:**
  Ensure the workout area is free of hazards that could lead to falls or injuries. Use supportive footwear and, if necessary, have stability aids (like a chair for balance exercises) available. The area should be well-lit, have enough space for movement, and be equipped with any necessary exercise equipment.

II.   During Workouts:

❖ Warm-Up and Cool-Down:
Incorporating a proper warm-up and cool-down into every workout session helps prepare the body for exercise and reduce the risk of injury. Warm-up exercises should gently raise the heart rate and warm up the muscles, while cool-down exercises should help gradually lower the heart rate and stretch the muscles.

❖ Hydration:
Staying hydrated is essential, especially for seniors, as they may have a diminished sense of thirst. Drinking water before, during, and after exercise helps prevent dehydration and maintain performance.

❖ Monitoring Intensity:
Seniors should be mindful of the intensity of their workouts. Using the "talk test" (being able to hold a conversation during exercise) can help gauge if the intensity level is appropriate. Additionally, heart rate monitors can be a useful tool for those who need to stay within a specific heart rate zone.

III.   After Workouts:

❖ Stretching:
Engaging in stretching exercises after a workout can improve flexibility and reduce muscle stiffness. Focus on major muscle groups and any areas that were particularly worked during the session.

❖ Nutrition:

Post-workout nutrition is important for recovery. Seniors should focus on consuming a balanced meal or snack that includes protein to aid muscle repair and carbohydrates to replenish energy stores.

❖ Rest and Recovery:

Adequate rest between workout sessions is essential for the body to recover and for muscle tissue to repair and strengthen. Seniors should listen to their bodies and allow for rest days, especially if experiencing soreness or fatigue.

By addressing these specific needs before, during, and after workouts, seniors can safely enjoy the multitude of benefits that regular physical activity offers, from improved mobility and strength to enhanced mental well-being.

Consulting with Healthcare Providers or Other Professionals Before Starting

Before embarking on a new workout regimen, consulting with healthcare providers or fitness professionals is a critical first step for seniors. This conversation ensures that the exercise plan is safe, effective, and tailored to individual health conditions and fitness levels. Here's what you need to communicate to your doctor, trainer, or physical therapist before starting your workouts:

I.   Medical History and Current Health Status:

❖ Chronic Conditions:

Inform them about any chronic conditions such as heart disease, diabetes, arthritis, or high blood pressure. These conditions can influence the type of exercises recommended and the intensity level.

❖ Medications:

Share a list of medications, including over-the-counter drugs and supplements. Some medications can affect your heart rate, blood pressure, and hydration levels during exercise.

❖ Previous Injuries or Surgeries:

Disclose any past injuries or surgeries, especially those that could affect your mobility or exercise capacity, such as joint replacements or back surgeries.

❖ Symptoms:

Discuss any symptoms you might be experiencing, such as chest pain, shortness of breath, dizziness, or joint pain. These symptoms could be important indicators of how to structure your workout plan.

II.   Fitness Level and Lifestyle:

❖ Current Activity Level:
Be honest about your current level of physical activity. This information helps in creating a starting point that is neither too easy nor overly challenging.

❖ Daily Routine:
Your daily routine can provide insights into your stamina, flexibility, and current physical challenges, helping tailor a workout plan that fits into your lifestyle.

❖ Goals:
Clearly articulate your fitness goals, whether it's improving balance, strengthening muscles, losing weight, or enhancing overall cardiovascular health. Goals help focus your workout plan.

III.   Preferences and Concerns:

❖ Exercise Preferences:
Discuss types of activities you enjoy or are interested in trying. Enjoyment is a key factor in sticking with an exercise program.

❖ Fears and Concerns:
If you have any fears or concerns about starting an exercise routine, such as the fear of falling or aggravating an old injury, bring these up. Addressing these concerns upfront can help in designing a program that feels safe and achievable.

IV.   Questions for Your Provider:

❖ Specific Recommendations:
Ask for specific exercise recommendations, including types of exercise to avoid and any modifications for your condition.

❖ Signs to Watch For:
Inquire about any signs or symptoms that should prompt you to stop exercising and seek medical advice.

❖ Follow-Up:
Discuss how often you should check in with them to update your exercise plan based on your progress or any changes in your health status.

By providing detailed information and asking the right questions, you can work with healthcare providers and fitness professionals to create a safe, effective workout plan tailored to your needs and goals. This collaborative approach ensures that you embark on your fitness journey with confidence, supported by expert advice tailored to your health profile.

Medication:	Dosage:	Date started taking:	Side effects noted:

Also, make a handwritten list of specific questions and list out all previous conditions, surgeries, and family history.

Safety First & Preventing Injuries

Safety First & Preventing Injuries

For seniors over 50 & 60, prioritizing safety and injury prevention is crucial before, during, and after workouts to ensure a healthy and sustainable exercise routine. Before beginning any new workout program, it's essential to get a comprehensive health check-up. Consulting with a healthcare provider can help identify any underlying health conditions that might affect the ability to exercise safely. It's also important to choose exercises that are suitable for one's current fitness level, potentially starting with lighter, more moderate activities and gradually increasing intensity based on comfort and ability. Pre-workout preparation should include a thorough warm-up to gently prepare the body for exercise, increasing blood flow to the muscles and reducing the risk of strains or sprains.

During workouts, maintaining proper form is key to preventing injuries. Seniors should be particularly mindful of their body's signals, avoiding pushing through pain or discomfort, which could indicate potential harm. Utilizing supportive equipment, like sturdy shoes and exercise mats, can also provide additional protection. Post-exercise, it's equally important to cool down with gentle stretching to aid in recovery and flexibility, helping to minimize post-workout soreness and stiffness. Hydration throughout the workout process cannot be overstated, as staying adequately hydrated supports overall health and helps prevent heat-related issues. By adhering to these guidelines and making safety a paramount concern, seniors can enjoy the vast benefits of physical activity while minimizing the risk of injury.

Understanding and Preventing Fall Risks

It's a startling reality, but falls are not an inevitable part of aging. Instead, they're often the result of a perfect storm: personal health issues meeting less-than-ideal environments. To stand tall against this, we dive deep into identifying both personal and environmental risk factors. From muscle weakness to cluttered living spaces, we're uncovering it all. But knowledge is only half the battle; action takes the victory. We lay out practical, straightforward steps to fortify your surroundings and yourself against falls. This includes creating a safe exercise area, free from hazards that could trip you up. Moreover, empowerment blooms through education—knowing how to fall safely and rise again is invaluable. This section is not just about avoiding falls; it's about building the confidence to move freely and fearlessly.

The Importance of Warm-Ups and Cool-Downs

Why do we start a car and let it idle a bit before hitting the road on a cold morning? The same principle applies to our bodies, especially as we age. Warm-ups and cool-downs are the bookends of a safe workout routine, ensuring our bodies are primed to move and then gently brought back to rest. Here, we explain the physiological magic behind these practices—increased blood flow, reduced injury risk, and a body that's ready to perform or recover. We don't just tell; we show. This section is packed with simple, effective routines that you can follow to ensure your body is warmed up properly before exercise and cooled down correctly afterward. It's about respecting your body's need for a gentle start and a gradual stop, turning injury prevention into a daily ritual.

Recognizing Your Body's Signals: When to Push and When to Pause

Our bodies communicate with us constantly, but understanding what they're saying is an art—especially when it comes to differentiating the discomfort of growth from the warning signs of potential injury. This chapter is your guide to interpreting these signals. We discuss the importance of recognizing when muscle soreness signifies progress and when it may indicate that you've pushed too far. Moreover, the role of rest days cannot be overstated; they're as crucial to your fitness journey as the workouts themselves, allowing for recovery and growth. Adjusting workouts in real-time, based on what your body tells you, is not just smart; it's essential for safe, effective exercise. And when in doubt, we underscore the importance of seeking professional medical advice, ensuring that your path to fitness is both ambitious and prudent. Remember, the goal is progress, not pain. Let's learn to listen, adapt, and thrive.

Sources:

httsps://www.cdc.gov/physicalactivity/basics/older_adults/index.htm

https://www.moradaseniorliving.com/senior-living-blog/debunking-6-myths-about-exercising-in-your-senior-years-when-aging-at-alsuma-ok-senior-independentfacility/#:~:text=It's%20a%20common%20misconception%20that,muscle%20mass%2C%20and%20enhance%20flexibility.

https://www.health.harvard.edu/staying-healthy/exercise-and-aging-can-you-walk-away-from-father-time

https://www.humangood.org/resources/senior-living-blog/low-impact-exercises-for-older-adults

Chapter 2

Building a Foundation: Core and Balance

Core Strengthening for Stability and Posture

At the heart of our bodily functions and movements is the core—a robust foundation that does more than just flaunt a six-pack. Understanding the anatomy of the core is crucial, as these muscles play a pivotal role in our stability, posture, and overall health. This section introduces safe, effective exercises tailored for seniors, designed to fortify the core, thereby enhancing stability and straightening our stance in the world. Beyond exercises, we delve into how a strengthened core can dramatically improve posture and alleviate back pain, offering practical tips for weaving core work seamlessly into your daily routines. It's about transforming mundane activities into opportunities for strength, one core-engaging moment at a time.

Core Strengthening for Stability and Posture Exercises

Strengthening the core is essential for seniors, as it directly impacts stability, balance, and posture, reducing the risk of falls and improving overall mobility. Here are 10 detailed core-strengthening workouts designed for seniors, focusing on safety and effectiveness. Before beginning any new exercise routine, consult with a healthcare provider to ensure these exercises are appropriate for your individual health status.

I.   Seated Marches:

* Sit upright on a chair with your feet flat on the ground.

* Engage your core muscles and lift your right knee towards your chest, then lower it

* Repeat with your left knee, alternating legs for 10-15 repetitions on each side.

* Keep your back straight and use your abdominal muscles to lift your legs

II.   Pelvic Tilts:

* Lie on your back with knees bent and feet flat on the floor, hip-width apart.

* Tighten your stomach muscles, pushing your lower back into the floor.

* Hold for 3-5 seconds, then relax.

* Perform 10-15 repetitions, ensuring smooth, controlled movements.

III.   Seated Leg Lifts:

* Sit on the edge of a chair with your legs extended in front, heels on the ground.

* Keeping your back straight, engage your core and lift leg at a time off the floor.

* Hold the lift for a few seconds, then lower back down gently.

* Do 10 repetitions on each leg, keeping the movements controlled.

IV.   Cat-Cow Stretch (Modified for Chair):

* Sit on a chair with your feet flat on the ground, hands on your knees.

* Inhale, arch your back, and look up towards the ceiling (Cow position).

* Exhale, round your spine, and tuck your chin to your chest (Cat position).

* Move between these two positions for 10-15 cycles, focusing on flexing and extending the spine.

V.   Bird Dog (Modified):

* Start on all fours on a mat, with knees under hips and hands under shoulders.

* Extend your right arm forward and your left leg back, keeping your body in a straight line from fingertips to toes.

* Hold for 3-5 seconds, then switch sides.

* Perform 8-10 repetitions on each side, maintaining balance and stability.

VI.   Side Bends:

* Stand with feet hip-width apart, or sit upright in a chair.

* Place one hand behind your head and the other arm by your side.

- ❖ Bend to the side opposite the hand behind your head, feeling a stretch along side.

- ❖ Return to the starting position and repeat on the other side.

- ❖ Do 10-15 bends on each side, keeping movements slow and controlled.

VII. Seated Russian Twists:

- ❖ Sit on the edge of a chair with feet flat on the ground.

- ❖ Lean back slightly, keeping your spine straight, and engage your core.

- ❖ Twist your torso to the right, then to the left, to complete one repetition.

- ❖ Perform 10-15 repetitions on each side, moving with control.

VIII. Bridge Lifts:

- ❖ Lie on your back with knees bent and feet flat on the floor, arms by your sides.

- ❖ Lift your hips towards the ceiling, squeezing your glutes at the top.

- ❖ Lower back down slowly to complete one repetition.

- ❖ Do 10-15 repetitions, focusing on engaging your core and glutes.

IX.   Plank (Modified for Seniors):

* Begin in a tabletop position on a mat.

* Step your feet back to form a straight line from head to heels, supporting on your knees instead of your toes for a modified version.

* Hold for 15-30 seconds, keeping your core engaged and your body in a straight line.

* Ensure your shoulders are directly over your wrists.

X.   Standing Knee Lifts:

* Stand behind a chair, lightly holding onto it for support.

* Slowly lift one knee towards your chest while keeping your core engaged.

* Lower the leg back down and repeat with the other leg.

* Do 10-15 repetitions on each leg, focusing on maintaining stability and posture.

Incorporate these exercises into your routine 2-3 times a week, paying attention to your body's signals and modifying as needed to accommodate your fitness level and mobility.

Balance Workouts That Reduce Fall Risk

As the years roll by, maintaining balance becomes a subtle art—a skill that, when honed, can significantly reduce the risk of falls. We start with the basics, shedding light on why balance might wane with age and how targeted exercises can counteract this trend. Follow our step-by-step guide to balance training exercises specifically curated for seniors, complete with methods to track your balance improvement journey. Furthermore, we reveal how everyday activities, when approached with intent, can serve as a platform for enhancing balance, turning every step into a conscious act of stability.

Balance Workouts That Reduce Fall Risk Exercises

Balance exercises are crucial for seniors to minimize the risk of falls and maintain independence. Here are 10 detailed balance workouts designed to enhance stability and reduce the risk of falls, emphasizing gradual progression and safety.

I. Single-Leg Stand

- Stand behind a chair or next to a wall for support.
- Shift your weight to one foot and lift the other foot slightly off the ground.
- Hold this position for 10-30 seconds, then switch legs.
- Focus on maintaining an upright posture throughout the exercise.

II. Heel-to-Toe Walk:

- Place the heel of one foot directly in front of the toes of the opposite foot as if walking on a tightrope.
- Take 10-15 steps forward in a heel-to-toe fashion.
- Extend your arms to the sides if you need extra balance.

III. Side Leg Raises:

- Stand behind a chair or next to a wall for support.

❖ Keep your body straight and lift one leg to the side, keeping the toe pointed forward.

❖ Hold the position for a few seconds, then lower the leg back down.

❖ Perform 10-15 repetitions on each side.

IV. Back Leg Raises:

❖ Stand behind a chair or next to a wall for support.

❖ Slowly lift one leg straight back without bending the knee or pointing the toes.

❖ Hold for a few seconds, then lower the leg.

❖ Do 10-15 repetitions on each side.

V. Standing March:

❖ Stand straight with feet hip-width apart.

❖ Lift your knees up one at a time, as if marching in place.

❖ Keep your back straight and use the chair or wall for support if needed.

❖ Continue for 1-2 minutes, focusing on control and balance.

VI. Tandem Stand:

❖ Stand with one foot directly in front of the other, heel to toe, as if on a balance beam.

❖ Hold onto a chair or wall for support if needed.

❖   Hold the position for 10-30 seconds, then switch the position of your feet and repeat.

VII.   Chair Squats:

❖ Stand in front of a chair with feet hip-width apart.

❖ Slowly lower your body as if to sit, bending at the hips and knees, then stop just above the chair before standing back up.

❖ Use your arms for balance and perform 10-15 repetitions.

VIII.   Clock Reach:

❖ Imagine standing in the center of a clock. With the left hand on a chair for support, lift your right leg and point to 12 o'clock, then to 3, 6, and 9 o'clock.

❖ Switch legs and hands to complete the exercise on the other side.

Repeat the sequence 5 times on each side.

IX.   Tai Chi Basics:

❖ Start with simple Tai Chi movements like "wave hands like clouds" by standing with feet shoulder-width apart and gently transferring weight from one leg to the other while moving your hands across your body.

❖ Focus on fluid movements and balance.

Balance Transfer:

- ❖ Stand and transfer your weight slowly from your toes to your heels and side to side.

- ❖ Perform this weight-shifting exercise for 1-2 minutes, keeping movements controlled and deliberate.

For all exercises, maintain a slow, controlled pace to maximize safety and effectiveness. Incorporate these balance workouts into your routine 2-3 times per week, gradually increasing difficulty as your balance improves. Always consult with a healthcare provider before starting a new exercise program, especially if you have concerns about your balance or risk of falling.

Incorporating Balance into Everyday Activities

The concept of functional fitness takes center stage here, emphasizing the integration of balance and core strength into daily life activities. Through mindful movement—be it standing, walking, or bending—we explore how to naturally boost balance, making every action a deliberate practice in stability. This section also provides invaluable tips for arranging your living space to support balance-enhancing activities safely, alongside suggesting hobbies that, while enjoyable, also contribute to your core and balance goals. It's about finding equilibrium in every aspect of life, from the ground up.

Incorporating Balance into Everyday Activities Exercises

Incorporating balance exercises into your daily routine can significantly enhance stability and reduce the risk of falls. Here are 10 practical examples of how to weave balanced workouts into your everyday activities, making them a seamless part of your lifestyle.

I.   **Brushing Teeth Balance:**

   ❖ Stand on one foot while brushing your teeth, switching feet halfway through. Use the bathroom counter for support if needed. This daily routine helps improve balance and strengthens leg muscles.

II.   **Cooking Flamingo:**

   ❖ While waiting for water to boil or food to cook, stand on one leg, mimicking a flamingo stance. Alternate legs every minute to work on balance. Hold onto the kitchen counter if necessary for stability.

III.   **Heel-Toe Walking in Line:**

   ❖ As you walk down a hallway or between rooms in your home, practice walking heel-to-toe, as if on a tightrope. This activity enhances coordination and balance with each step.

IV.   **Standing from a Chair without Hands:**

   ❖ When getting up from a chair, try to stand up without using your hands. This movement strengthens your legs and core, improving your ability to balance during transitions.

V.   Calf Raises While Washing Dishes:

* ❖ While standing at the sink, perform calf raises by lifting your heels off the ground and then lowering them. This exercise can help strengthen the lower leg muscles, contributing to better balance.

VI.   Single-Leg Stand While Waiting:

* ❖ Anytime you find yourself standing and waiting, lift one foot off the ground and balance on the other leg. Whether you're in line at the store or waiting for a bus, this is a practical way to incorporate balance training.

VII.   Sitting to Standing Without Using Hands:

* ❖ Practice sitting down in a chair and standing back up without using your hands. Start by pushing up from the chair with your legs until you're able to do it without any momentum, focusing on controlled movements to enhance core strength and balance.

VIII.   Laundry Basket Squats:

* ❖ When lifting a laundry basket, squat instead of bending at the waist. Keep the basket close to your body, engage your core, and focus on keeping your balance as you squat and stand. This functional movement strengthens your legs and improves stability.

IX.   Balance on a Cushion:

* ❖ While doing tasks like folding laundry, stand on a cushion or a soft surface to challenge your balance. This subtle change can engage your core and leg muscles differently, improving your balance over time.

X.   Tiptoe Reaches:

❖ When reaching for items on high shelves, go onto your
   tiptoes instead of stretching. This not only helps with
   reaching items safely but also works on your balance and
   strengthens calf muscles.

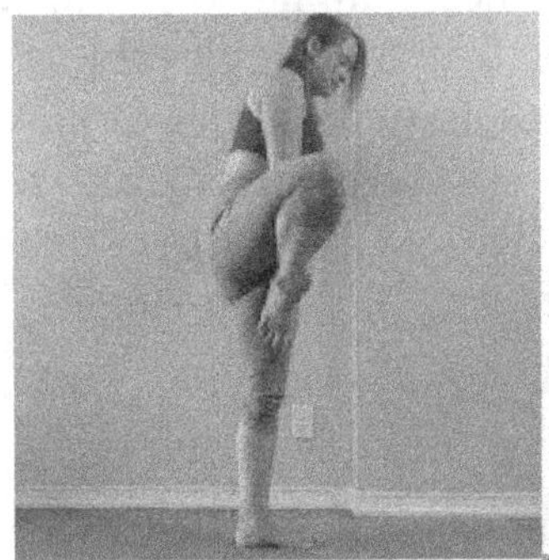

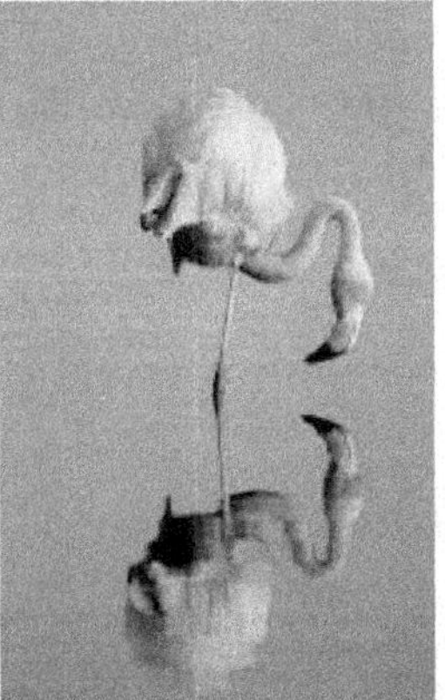

While waiting for water to boil or food to cook, stand on one leg, mimicking a flamingo stance.
Alternate legs every minute to work on balance. Hold onto the kitchen counter if necessary for
stability.

Incorporating these balance-enhancing activities into your daily
routines can significantly improve your stability and reduce the
risk of falls. Remember, consistency is key, and integrating balance
exercises into everyday tasks makes it easier to maintain a
balanced and healthy lifestyle.

29

Fun Balance Challenges to Do with Friends Exercises

Fitness, particularly when it comes to balance, doesn't have to be a solitary journey. Exercising with friends or in groups not only elevates motivation but also injects joy into the pursuit of health. Here, we explore the social side of balance training, offering a plethora of group activities and exercises that are as enjoyable as they are beneficial. From navigating community resources to kick starting your own senior fitness group, this section is a call to action to join forces with peers. Together, you'll discover that improving balance can be a shared adventure, filled with laughter, camaraderie, and the collective triumph of standing strong, side by side.

Incorporating balance challenges into social activities can make improving your stability both enjoyable and effective. Here are 10 fun balance exercises and challenges that you can do with friends, encouraging camaraderie and a bit of healthy competition.

I. **Partner Stand-Up:**

- ❖ Sit back-to-back with a friend on the ground with your knees bent.

- ❖ Try to stand up together without using your hands, relying on balance and teamwork.

- ❖ This challenge strengthens your core and enhances coordination.

II. **Tandem Walking Race:**

- ❖ Mark a straight line or use a balance beam if available.

- ❖ Walk heel-to-toe along the line as fast as you can, but if you step off, you must go back to the start.

- ❖ Race against a friend or take turns timing each other for the fastest walk without losing balance.

III.   Mirror Movements:

- ❖ Stand facing each other. One person leads by performing various balance exercises (e.g., leg stands, arm raises) while the other person tries to mirror them exactly.

- ❖ This not only tests balance but also reaction time and coordination.

IV.   Pass the Ball:

- ❖ Stand in a circle with friends, all balancing on one leg.

- ❖ Pass a ball around the circle without letting your lifted foot touch the ground.

- ❖ If someone drops the ball or loses balance, they're out. Last person balancing wins.

V.   Balance Tag:

- ❖ Play a game of tag where everyone must be balancing on one leg.

- ❖ If you put your foot down or switch legs, you're "it."

This adds a fun challenge to maintaining balance under dynamic conditions.

VI.   Yoga Pose Competition:

- ❖ Take turns choosing a yoga pose that involves balance (e.g., Tree Pose, Warrior III).

❖ Everyone attempts the pose, and the last person to hold it without falling or breaking form wins the round.

VII.   Stability Ball Toss:

❖ Sit on stability balls a short distance apart and toss a lightweight ball or balloon back and forth.

❖ Try to keep your balance on the ball without letting your feet move from their spot.

VIII.   Blindfolded Balance:

❖ Stand on one leg with a blindfold on, and have a friend time you.

❖ See who can balance the longest without sight. Removing visual cues significantly increases the challenge.

IX.   Obstacle Course:

❖ Set up a simple obstacle course that includes balance challenges, such as walking on a narrow path, stepping over objects, and balancing on cushions.

❖ Navigate the course with a friend timing each other, adding playful penalties for losing balance.

X.   Freeze Dance Balance:

❖ Play music and dance around, but when the music stops, everyone must freeze in a balance challenging position.

❖ The last person to successfully hold their pose without moving or falling wins.

These activities not only help improve balance but also build stronger relationships through shared experiences and support. Remember, the goal is to have fun and challenge each other while staying safe. Always adapt activities to fit the fitness levels of all participants to ensure everyone can join in the fun.

Sources:

https://www.health.harvard.edu/staying-healthy/the-best-core-exercises-for-older-adults

https://www.goodrx.com/health-topic/senior-health/balance-exercises-for-seniors

https://www.eehealth.org/blog/2022/02/chair-exercises-for-limited-mobility/

 https://www.ncbi.nlm.nih.gov/pmc/articles/PMC6304477/

ChatGPT4.0   (2024,   January   18)   Retrieved   from [https://chat.openai.com].

Chapter 3

Gaining Strength and Flexibility

Strength Training: Resistance Bands and Bodyweight Exercises

Strength training isn't just for the young and the restless; it's a cornerstone of maintaining vitality at any age, especially for seniors. It bolsters bone health, boosts your metabolism, and builds the muscle mass that age tries to take away. Enter resistance bands and bodyweight exercises—your allies in this fight against the clock. Resistance bands offer a low-impact, highly effective method to build strength safely. Coupled with bodyweight exercises, they form a dynamic duo that enhances muscle strength without the need for heavy equipment. This section not only guides you through getting started with these tools but also how to weave them into a balanced routine, ensuring your strength training is as comprehensive as it is enjoyable.

Strength Training: Resistance Bands and Bodyweight Exercises

Integrating resistance bands and bodyweight exercises into your routine can significantly improve strength, flexibility, and overall fitness. Here are 10 detailed workouts combining both methods, designed to target major muscle groups and enhance functional strength.

❑ **Resistance Band Squats:**

* Stand on a resistance band with feet shoulder-width apart, holding the ends with both hands at shoulder level.

* Lower into a squat while keeping the band under tension, then rise back up to the starting position.

* Perform 10-15 repetitions, ensuring your knees don't extend past your toes during the squat.

❑ **Push-Ups:**

* Begin in a plank position with your hands slightly wider than shoulder-width apart.

* Lower your body towards the ground, keeping your elbows close to your body, then push back up to the starting position.

* Modify by dropping to your knees if needed. Aim for 8-12 repetitions.

❑ **Resistance Band Rows:**

* Sit on the floor with legs extended, wrap a resistance band around your feet, and hold the ends in each hand.

  Pull the band towards your waist, squeezing your shoulder blades together, then slowly release.

* Complete 10-15 repetitions, maintaining a straight back throughout the exercise.

❑ **Glute Bridges:**

❖ Lie on your back with knees bent and feet flat on the floor, hip-width apart.

❖ Lift your hips towards the ceiling, squeezing your glutes at the top, then lower back down.

❖ For added resistance, place a resistance band above your knees. Perform 10-15 repetitions.

❑ **Standing Resistance Band Bicep Curls:**

❖ Stand in the middle of a resistance band, holding the ends in each hand with palms facing forward.

❖ Curl your hands towards your shoulders, keeping your elbows stationary, then lower back down.

❖ Do 10-15 repetitions, keeping the movement controlled.

❑ **Tricep Dips:**

❖ Use a stable chair or bench. Sit on the edge with your hands next to your hips.

❖ Slide your hips off the chair, supporting your weight with your arms.

❖ Lower your body by bending your elbows, then press back up.

❖ Complete 8-12 repetitions, keeping your elbows pointed back.

❑ **Resistance Band Lateral Walks:**

❖ Place a resistance band just above your knees and stand with feet shoulder-width apart, in a slight squat position.

❖ Step to the side in a controlled manner, then step back in the opposite direction.

❖ Perform 10-15 steps in each direction, keeping tension on the band.

❑ **Plank:**

❖ Hold a plank position from your hands (or forearms) and toes, with your body in a straight line from head to heels.

❖ Engage your core and glutes to keep your hips stable. Hold for 30 seconds to 1 minute.

❖ To modify, plank from your knees while maintaining a straight line through your body.

❑ **Resistance Band Chest Press:**

❖ Wrap a resistance band behind your back, holding the ends with both hands at chest

❖ Press your arms straight out in front of you, then slowly return to the starting position.

❖ Perform 10-15 repetitions, keeping your movements smooth and controlled.

❑ **Bodyweight Lunges:**

❖ Stand with feet hip-width apart. Step forward with one leg and lower your hips until both knees are bent at about a 90-degree angle.

❖ Make sure your front knee is directly above your ankle.

❖ Push back up to the starting position. Alternate legs, performing 10-15 lunges on each side.

These exercises offer a comprehensive approach to strength training that can be adapted to various fitness levels. Always start with lighter resistance or fewer repetitions, gradually increasing as your strength improves. Remember to maintain good form and breathe consistently throughout each exercise.

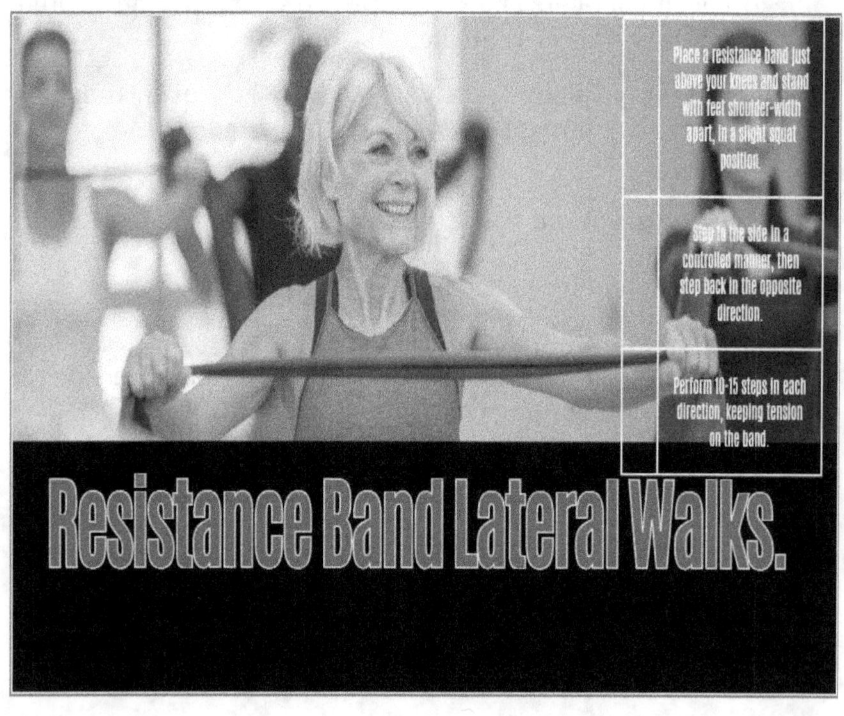

Flexibility Moves for Every Muscle

Flexibility: the unsung hero of physical fitness, especially as we age. It's what keeps us agile, ensures our movements are fluid, and significantly lowers our risk of injuries. Here, we dive into the art and science of stretching—showing you techniques to enhance flexibility across every muscle group. From the basics of stretching to targeted stretches designed with seniors in mind, this chapter is a comprehensive guide to making flexibility a pillar of your fitness regimen. By integrating these exercises into your daily routine, you're not just reaching for your toes; you're reaching for a life where every move is easier and every day is more comfortable.

Flexibility Moves for Every Muscle Exercises

Improving flexibility is crucial for overall mobility, injury prevention, and can enhance performance in physical activities. Here are 10 detailed stretching exercises designed to target major muscle groups and improve flexibility across the entire body. Each stretch should be held for 15-30 seconds, repeated 2-3 times, and performed when the muscles are warm, such as after a workout or a warm bath.

- **Neck Stretch:**

  - ❖ Sit or stand with good posture.

  - ❖ Gently tilt your head toward one shoulder until you feel a stretch along the side of your neck.

  - ❖ Hold, then slowly lift your head back to the center and repeat on the other side.

❏ **Shoulder Stretch:**

❖ Bring one arm across your body.

❖ Use the other hand to press the arm closer to your chest, stretching the shoulder.

❖ Hold, then switch arms.

❏ **Triceps Stretch:**

❖ Raise one arm overhead, bend the elbow, and reach your hand down towards the opposite shoulder blade.

❖ Use your other hand to gently push on the bent elbow for a deeper stretch.

❖ Hold, then switch arms.

❏ **Chest Stretch:**

❖ Stand in a doorway or against a wall.

❖ Place your arm against the wall at shoulder height, elbow bent at 90 degrees.

❖ Gently turn your body away from the wall until you feel a stretch across your chest and shoulder.

❖ Hold, then switch sides.

❏ **Upper Back Stretch:**

❖ Sit or stand with arms extended in front of you.

- ❖ Clasp your hands together, round your back, and push your hands forward.

- ❖ Lower your head between your arms to feel the stretch in your upper back.

☐ **Cat-Cow Stretch:**

- ❖ Start on all fours with hands under shoulders and knees under hips.

- ❖ Inhale, arch your back (cow), lifting your head and tailbone.

- ❖ Exhale, round your spine (cat), tucking your chin to your chest.

- ❖ Continue to flow between these two positions.

☐ **Seated Hamstring Stretch:**

- ❖ Sit on the floor with one leg extended and the other bent, foot against the inner thigh of the extended leg

- ❖ Lean forward from your hips over the extended leg, keeping your back straight.

- ❖ Hold, then switch legs.

□ **Quadriceps Stretch:**

❖ Stand and hold onto a chair or wall for balance.

❖ Bend one knee and bring your heel towards your buttock, holding your ankle with your hand.

❖ Keep your knees together and push your hip forward to feel the stretch in the front of your thigh.

❖ Hold, then switch legs.

□ **Calf Stretch:**

❖ Stand arm's length from a wall.

❖ Step one foot back, keeping it straight, and press the heel into the floor.

❖ Bend your front knee, keeping both heels on the ground, until you feel a stretch in the back leg's calf

❖ Hold, then switch legs.

□ **Seated Hip and Glute Stretch:**

❖ Sit on a chair and cross one ankle over the opposite knee, creating a "figure 4."

❖ Gently lean forward while keeping your back straight, pressing your crossed knee down to intensify the stretch.

❖ Hold, then switch sides.

Performing these stretches regularly can significantly improve your flexibility, reduce stiffness, and contribute to a more comfortable and active lifestyle. Remember to stretch gently and avoid bouncing, which can cause muscle strain.

Low-Impact Cardio Options for Strength and Endurance Exercises

Low-impact cardio exercises are ideal for seniors looking to improve cardiovascular health, strength, and endurance without putting excessive stress on the joints. Here are 10 detailed low-impact cardio workouts designed to be effective and safe for seniors.

I.   Brisk Walking:

- ❖ A simple yet effective low-impact cardio exercise. Aim for a brisk pace that elevates your heart rate.

- ❖ Integrate intervals by walking faster for 1 minute, then at a normal pace for 2 minutes.

- ❖ Repeat for 20-30 minutes.

II.   Aqua Aerobics:

- ❖ Water provides natural resistance and supports the body, reducing the risk of injury.

- ❖ Join an aqua aerobics class or perform exercises like leg lifts, arm circles, and walking or jogging in place in the water for 30 minutes.

III.   Cycling on a Stationary Bike:

- ❖ Adjust the seat height to ensure minimal stress on your knees.

❖ Cycle at a moderate pace for 20-30 minutes, varying the resistance to include some intervals for increased intensity.

IV.   Elliptical Trainer:

❖ Use an elliptical machine to simulate walking or running with reduced impact.

❖ Maintain a steady pace for 20-30 minutes, optionally using the arm levers to engage the upper body.

V.   Dance Fitness Classes:

❖ Participate in a dance fitness class geared towards seniors, focusing on low-impact movements.

❖ Enjoy the social aspect and the variety of music and dance styles for 30-60 minutes.

VI.   Tai Chi:

❖ Practice Tai Chi, a form of martial arts known for its health benefits and low impact movements.

❖ Join a class or follow a video at home, focusing on fluid movements and balance for 30-60 minutes.

VII.   Yoga for Cardio:

❖ Although not traditionally viewed as cardio, dynamic yoga styles (like Vinyasa) can elevate the heart rate.

❖ Practice a flow sequence that includes sun salutations and standing poses for 30- 60 minutes.

VIII. Step Aerobics:

- ❖ Engage in a low-impact step aerobics class, using a step platform.

- ❖ Perform steps and sequences at a pace that's comfortable for you, for 20-30 minutes.

IX. Nordic Walking:

- ❖ Use walking poles to engage the upper body while walking at a brisk pace.

- ❖ The poles help distribute your weight and reduce impact on the knees and ankles.

Walk for 30-60 minutes.

X. Gentle Kickboxing:

- ❖ Join a class or follow a video that modifies kickboxing moves to be low impact.

- ❖ Focus on controlled movements, punches, and kicks without jumping, for 20-30 minutes.

Incorporating these low-impact cardio exercises into your routine can significantly improve your cardiovascular health, endurance, and overall well-being, all while keeping joint stress to a minimum. Always start with a warm-up and conclude with a cool-down to prevent injuries. Adjust the intensity and duration to match your current fitness level and consult with a healthcare provider before starting a new exercise program.

Pilates for Seniors: Strengthening and Lengthening Exercises

Pilates is an excellent exercise regimen for seniors, focusing on core strength, flexibility, balance, and overall body awareness. Here are 11 Pilates exercises tailored for seniors, designed to strengthen and lengthen muscles without overstraining.

I.   Pelvic Tilts:

- Lie on your back with knees bent and feet flat on the floor.

- Slowly tilt your pelvis towards you, flattening your lower back against the floor.

- Hold for 3 seconds, then gently return to the starting position.

- Perform 10 repetitions.

II.   Foot Circles:

- Lie on your back with one leg extended straight up, perpendicular to the floor. The other leg can be bent with the foot flat on the ground or extended flat for more challenge.

- Circle your raised foot slowly, keeping the movement controlled from the hip.

- Do 5 circles in each direction, then switch legs.

III.   Leg Slide:

- Lie on your back with knees bent, feet flat on the floor.

- Slowly slide one leg out until it's straight, then slide it back in.

❖ Keep your pelvis stable and engaged throughout the movement.

❖ Perform 8-10 repetitions on each leg.

IV.   Arm Reaches:

❖ Sit or stand with your spine in a neutral position.

❖ Extend your arms in front of you at shoulder height, then open them wide to the sides.

❖ Bring them back in front and repeat, focusing on keeping your shoulders down and back engaged.

❖ Do 10-15 repetitions.

V.   Spine Twist:

❖ Sit up tall on a chair or on the floor with legs crossed.

❖ Extend your arms out to the sides at shoulder height.

❖ Gently twist your torso to one side, leading with your head and shoulders. Keep your hips facing forward.

❖ Return to center and twist to the other side.

❖ Perform 5 twists to each side.

VI.   Seated Leg Lifts:

❖ Sit on the edge of a chair with your back straight.

❖ Extend one leg out straight at a diagonal, then lift it up as high as comfortable.

❖ Lower it back down without touching the floor and repeat.

❖ Do 8-10 lifts on each leg.

VII.   Cat-Cow Stretch:

❖ On all fours, align your wrists under your shoulders and your knees under your hips.

❖ Inhale, arch your back down while looking up (Cow).

❖ Exhale, round your spine up towards the ceiling while tucking your chin (Cat).

❖ Flow between these two positions for 8-10 cycles.

VIII.   The Hundred:

❖ Lie on your back with knees bent into your chest and head and shoulders lifted off the floor.

❖ Extend your arms by your sides, palms down. Extend legs to a 45-degree angle if possible.

❖ Pump your arms up and down in small movements, breathing in for 5 pumps and out for 5 pumps.

❖ Do this for a count of 100 pumps.

IX.   Side Leg Lifts:

❖ Lie on your side with legs extended, propping your head up with your hand or resting it on your arm.

❖ Lift your top leg towards the ceiling, then lower it with control.

❖ Keep your hips stacked and core engaged.

❖ Perform 8-10 lifts on each side.

X.   Mermaid Stretch:

- ❖ Sit with your legs folded to one side, knees bent.

- ❖ Place one hand on the floor beside you and reach the other arm over your head, stretching the side of your body.

- ❖ Hold for a few seconds, then switch sides.

- ❖ Do 5 stretches on each side.

XI.   Arm Circles:

- ❖ Lift both arms out to your sides, and keep them straight.

- ❖ This is your starting position.

- ❖ Move your arms in a forward circle 10 times.

- ❖ Move your arms in a backward circle 10 times.

- ❖ Repeat steps two and three at least three times.

These Pilates exercises are aimed at building strength and increasing flexibility in a gentle, low-impact manner suitable for seniors. Remember to move through each exercise with control and focus on your breath, which is a core principle of Pilates practice. Always consult with a professional before starting a new workout routine, especially if you have existing health concerns.

Sources:

https://www.cdc.gov/physicalactivity/downloads/growing_stronger.pdf

https://www.litmethod.com/blogs/boltcut-blog/resistance-band-exercises-for-seniors

https://www.humangood.org/resources/senior-living-blog/low-impact-exercises-for-older-adults

https://www.youtube.com/watch?v=kFhG-ZzLNN4

Chapter 4

Mind-Body Connection

The Basics of Tai Chi: Movement and Meditation and Exercises

Tai Chi, often described as meditation in motion, offers a unique blend of gentle physical activity and mental concentration. This ancient practice, with its roots steeped in martial arts, has evolved into a form of exercise that's especially beneficial for seniors, focusing on slow, deliberate movements paired with deep breathing. This section introduces you to the world of Tai Chi, highlighting its health benefits, which range from improved balance and reduced fall risk to enhanced mental well-being. We guide you through simple Tai Chi sequences that are accessible to beginners, emphasizing the importance of mindfulness and the connection between movement and breath. Additionally, we offer practical advice on finding Tai Chi classes tailored for seniors or tips for starting a practice at home, ensuring you have the tools to begin this transformative journey.

Tai Chi, an ancient Chinese martial art known for its health benefits, combines slow, deliberate movements with deep breathing and meditation. Here are 10 foundational Tai Chi exercises (often referred to as forms or movements) that introduce the basics of movement and meditation, suitable for beginners and particularly beneficial for seniors.

I. **Opening the Chest:**

- ❖ Stand with your feet shoulder-width apart and knees slightly bent.

- ❖ Breathe in and slowly raise your arms in front of you, palms up, to shoulder height.

- ❖ Exhale, opening your arms wide to the sides, expanding your chest.

- ❖ Inhale as you bring your arms back in front, exhale as you lower them to the sides.

- ❖ Repeat 8-10 times.

II. **Parting the Wild Horse's Mane**:

- ❖ From a standing position, step left with your left foot, shifting your weight forward.

- ❖ Simultaneously, raise your left arm up and forward as if gently parting through tall grass, while your right hand sweeps down and back.

- ❖ Return to the starting position and repeat on the opposite side.

- ❖ Perform 5 repetitions per side.

III. **Wave Hands Like Clouds:**

- ❖ Stand with your feet wider than shoulder-width. Keep your knees soft and your body relaxed.

- ❖ Hold your arms in front of you as if holding a ball. Gently shift your weight from side to side, turning your waist.

❖ As you turn, let your arms flow smoothly from side to side as if moving clouds through the sky. Continue for 1-2 minutes, focusing on fluidity and breath.

IV.   Golden Rooster Stands on One Leg:

❖ Begin in a neutral standing position. Focus on grounding yourself through your feet.

❖ Slowly transfer your weight to your left leg while inhaling and lifting your right knee up.

❖ Simultaneously, lift your right arm forward and up, and your left arm down and back for balance.

❖ Hold for a few breaths, then switch sides. Repeat 3-4 times on each side.

V.   Repulse the Monkey:

❖ Start with your feet shoulder-width apart and your knees slightly bent.

❖ Raise your right arm up to shoulder height, palm facing forward, as you step back with your left foot.

❖ Simultaneously, pull your right arm back like drawing a bow, turning your torso slightly to the right.

❖ Step forward again, and repeat on the other side, moving slowly and deliberately.

Do 5 repetitions per side.

VI.   Brush Knee and Push:

❖ Stand with your feet shoulder-width apart. Step forward with your left foot.

- ❖ Simultaneously, "brush" your left knee with your left hand while your right hand "pushes" forward, palms facing outward.

- ❖ Return to the starting position and repeat on the opposite side. Perform 5 repetitions per side.

VII.   Grasping the Bird's Tail:

- ❖ Begin in a standing position, stepping out to the left into a wide stance.

- ❖ Shift your weight to the left, extending your left arm in a ward-off position. Circle your right arm under your left, then push forward.

- ❖ Roll back, rotating your arms, and then push again. Switch sides after 5 repetitions.

VIII.   Stork Cools Its Wings:

- ❖ Stand with your feet together, then step slightly back with one foot.

- ❖ Raise both arms at the sides with elbows slightly bent, like the wings of a bird.

- ❖ Lean forward slightly from the hips, then slowly straighten up while lowering the arms.

- ❖ Perform 5 repetitions before switching the standing leg.

IX.   Needle at Sea Bottom:

- ❖ From a standing position, shift your weight to one leg.

* Lean forward slightly, extending one hand downwards as if to touch the sea bottom, while the other arm sweeps back for balance.

* Keep your back straight and avoid bending too far. Switch sides after 5 repetitions.

Closing Form:

* Stand with your feet shoulder-width apart, arms relaxed at your sides.

* Slowly raise your arms in front of you, palms down, as you inhale.

* Exhale and gently lower your arms, visualizing gathering tranquility and energy.

* Repeat the movement 3-5 times, focusing on the sensation of calming energy enveloping your body.

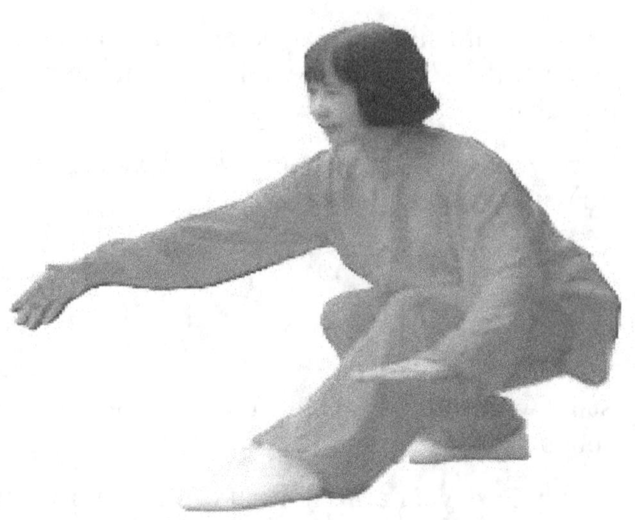

Needle Sea Bottom Tai Chi Pose

Practicing these Tai Chi forms promotes not only physical strength and flexibility but also mental clarity and stress reduction. Focus on the flow of movements and your breath, allowing a meditative state to enhance the overall experience. As you become more comfortable with these basics, you can explore more complex sequences and incorporate them into a longer practice.

Yoga for Mindfulness and Mobility and Exercises

Yoga combines physical postures, breathing techniques, and meditation to enhance both mental and physical well-being. Here are 10 detailed yoga workouts or examples designed to promote mindfulness and improve mobility, especially tailored for seniors.

Mountain Pose (Tadasana) with Deep Breathing:

- ❖ Stand tall with feet hip-width apart, arms at your sides.

- ❖ Inhale deeply, raising your arms overhead, palms facing each other.

- ❖ Exhale slowly, lowering your arms back to your sides.

- ❖ Repeat for 5 breath cycles, focusing on standing strong and steady.

Chair Pose (Utkatasana):

- ❖ From Mountain Pose, inhale and raise your arms straight above your head.

- ❖ Exhale and bend your knees, as if sitting back into an invisible chair.

- ❖ Hold for 3-5 breaths, focusing on maintaining balance and strength in your legs.

- ❖ Return to Mountain Pose.

Warrior II (Virabhadrasana II):

- ❖ Step your feet about 3-4 feet apart.

- ❖ Raise your arms parallel to the floor and turn your right foot out 90 degrees and your left foot in slightly.

- ❖ Bend your right knee, ensuring it's over your ankle, and gaze out over your right hand.

- ❖ Hold for 5 breaths, then switch sides.

Tree Pose (Vrksasana):

- ❖ Stand with your feet hip-width apart. Shift your weight onto your left foot.

- ❖ Place your right foot on your inner left thigh or calf (avoid the knee) and balance.

- ❖ Bring your palms together in front of your chest or raise them above your head.

- ❖ Hold for 5-8 breaths, then switch legs.

Seated Forward Bend (Paschimottanasana):

- ❖ Sit on the floor with your legs stretched out in front of you.

- ❖ Inhale and lengthen your spine.

- ❖ Exhale and gently fold forward from your hips, reaching for your feet or shins.

- ❖ Hold for 5-8 breaths, focusing on the stretch in your hamstrings and spine.

Cat-Cow Stretch (Marjaryasana-Bitilasana):

- ❖ Start on your hands and knees, with wrists under shoulders and knees under hips.

- ❖ Inhale, arch your back, and look up (Cow).

- ❖ Exhale, round your spine, and tuck your chin to your chest (Cat).

- ❖ Flow between these two poses for 1-2 minutes, synchronizing movement with breath.

Cobra Pose (Bhujangasana):

- ❖ Lie on your stomach with your hands under your shoulders and elbows close to your body.

- ❖ Inhale and gently lift your chest off the floor, using your back muscles.

- ❖ Hold for 3-5 breaths, focusing on opening your chest and shoulders.

- ❖ Exhale to gently lower back down.

Child's Pose (Balasana):

- ❖ From your hands and knees, sit back on your heels and fold forward, extending your arms in front of you.

- ❖ Rest your forehead on the floor and relax your entire body.

- ❖ Hold for 5-10 breaths, focusing on releasing tension in your back, shoulders, and arms.

Legs-Up-The-Wall Pose (Viparita Karani):

* ❖ Sit with one side of your body against a wall, then gently swing your legs up onto the wall as you lie back.

* ❖ Rest your arms at your sides or on your belly.

* ❖ Hold for 5-10 minutes, focusing on deep, relaxing breaths.

Corpse Pose (Savasana) with Guided Meditation:

* ❖ Lie flat on your back, legs slightly apart, arms at your sides with palms facing up.

* ❖ Close your eyes and take deep breaths, focusing on relaxing every part of your body from your toes to your head.

* ❖ Stay in this pose for 5-10 minutes, using this time to meditate or simply focus on your breath.

These yoga poses and practices are designed to enhance mindfulness and mobility, promoting a sense of calm and increasing flexibility. Always listen to your body, modifying poses as needed to suit your comfort level.

Breathing Techniques for Relaxation and Energy

Breathing techniques can play a pivotal role in enhancing both relaxation and energy levels, making them an essential component of a holistic approach to senior fitness and well-being. Two effective practices are diaphragmatic breathing for calming and relaxation, and Kapalbhati breathing for vitality and energy.

Diaphragmatic Breathing:

This technique focuses on deep, rhythmic breathing using the diaphragm rather than shallow chest breathing. It promotes relaxation by activating the body's natural relaxation response, reducing stress and anxiety levels.

How to Practice Diaphragmatic Breathing:

- ❖ Find a comfortable seated or lying position. Place one hand on your chest and the other on your abdomen.

- ❖ Slowly inhale through your nose, aiming to make the hand on your abdomen rise higher than the one on your chest. This indicates that the diaphragm is pulling air into the bases of your lungs.

- ❖ Pause for a moment at the top of your inhale.

- ❖ Exhale slowly through your mouth, feeling the hand on your abdomen lower as you engage your abdominal muscles, pushing the air out.

- ❖ Repeat this pattern for 5-10 minutes, focusing on slow, deep breaths that fill and empty your lungs fully.

Kapalbhati Breathing:

Kapalbhati, a form of pranayama found in yoga practice, is known for its energizing effects. It involves short, powerful exhales and passive inhales. This practice is thought to improve lung capacity, clear the nasal passages, and energize the mind.

How to Practice Kapalbhati Breathing:

- ❖ Sit in a comfortable position with your spine straight. Place your hands on your knees, palms facing up or in a mudra position.

❖ Take a deep breath in.

❖ Exhale forcefully through your nose by contracting your abdominal muscles quickly, then let your lungs fill naturally, without actively inhaling.

❖ Begin with a cycle of 10 such breaths, then gradually increase to two more rounds according to your comfort and capacity.

Both diaphragmatic and Kapalbhati breathing exercises offer distinct benefits and can be incorporated into daily routines. Diaphragmatic breathing is particularly beneficial for winding down or preparing for sleep, while Kapalbhati can serve as a morning energizer or a midday pick-me-up. However, it's important for seniors to approach Kapalbhati with caution, especially those with respiratory issues, high blood pressure, or hernias, consulting healthcare providers before practice. Integrating these breathing techniques can significantly contribute to improved mental and physical health, aiding relaxation and enhancing energy levels when practiced regularly.

Sources:

https://www.aegisliving.com/resource-center/the-health-benefits-of
-tai-chi-for-seniors/

https://www.silversneakers.com/blog/yoga-seniors-poses-improve-
balance/

https://www.kendalathome.org/blog/breathe-easy-six-breath-exerci
ses-for-older-adults

https://www.ncbi.nlm.nih.gov/pmc/articles/PMC4868399/

Do you like these workouts? Keep Reading more workouts ahead!
Please Leave a review.
https://amzn.to/3YQGbQO
Scan the QR code below to leave your review:

Chapter 5

Setting Realistic Goals and Tracking Progress

How to Set Achievable Fitness Goals

Success in fitness, especially for seniors, begins with setting goals that are not just ambitious but also realistic and personalized. This chapter guides you through defining what success looks like for you, taking into account your health status, lifestyle, and personal preferences. We introduce the SMART criteria—Specific, Measurable, Achievable, Relevant, Time-bound—as a framework for establishing fitness goals that are both inspiring and attainable. Emphasizing the need for balance, we discuss setting objectives that are challenging yet safe, incorporating both short-term achievements and long-term aspirations to keep you motivated and engaged on your fitness journey.

The Importance of Keeping an Exercise Journal

Keeping an exercise journal is a powerful tool for monitoring your progress, understanding patterns in your fitness routine, and recognizing the impact of exercise on your mood and physical well-being. This section explores different journaling methods, from traditional notebooks to digital apps, offering you options to find the format that best suits your preferences. We stress the importance of regularly reviewing your journal entries, not just as a record of what you've done but as a source of insight and inspiration, helping you adjust your goals and methods to better align with your evolving needs and preferences.

Celebrating Milestones and Adjusting Goals

Acknowledging your achievements, no matter how small, is crucial for maintaining motivation and commitment to your fitness journey. This chapter emphasizes the significance of celebrating milestones, suggesting healthy and fulfilling ways to reward yourself for reaching your goals. It also covers the importance of flexibility in goal setting, advising on how to adjust your objectives based on your progress and any new health considerations. The concept of continuous improvement is introduced, encouraging you to view your fitness journey as an evolving process, with goals that grow and change as you do.

Using Technology to Track Fitness Progress

Technology offers a myriad of ways to enhance and track your fitness progress, from apps that log your workouts to wearables that monitor your heart rate and activity levels. This section introduces various technological tools available to seniors, providing guidance on selecting devices that meet your needs and preferences. We also cover how to analyze the data collected by these tools to refine your fitness strategy, along with advice on managing privacy concerns and ensuring the safe use of technology in your fitness routine.

Staying Motivated: Tips and Tricks

Staying motivated can be challenging, but understanding the 'why' behind your fitness goals can help maintain your drive over the long term. This chapter offers strategies for sustaining motivation, including building a support network through online forums, local groups, or fitness classes, and introducing variety into your workouts to keep them engaging. Additionally, we explore the importance of maintaining a positive mindset, viewing setbacks as opportunities for learning and growth, and continuously seeking ways to enrich and diversify your fitness journey.

Sources:

https://health.clevelandclinic.org/smart-fitness-goals

https://smartwatchinsight.com/best-fitness-tracker-for-seniors/

https://www.nia.nih.gov/health/exercise-and-physical-activity/stayi
ng-motivated-exercise-tips-older-adults

Chapter 6

Exercises for Every Situation

<u>Creating an Effective Home Gym on a Budget</u>

Creating a home gym doesn't have to empty your pockets. This section introduces cost-effective, versatile equipment that can transform any corner of your home into a personal fitness studio. From resistance bands to stability balls, we highlight tools that offer maximum benefits without breaking the bank. Dive into DIY solutions, turning everyday household items into innovative exercise equipment for strength, balance, and flexibility workouts. Organize your workout area efficiently, even in limited spaces, and discover online resources offering free or affordable workout programs tailored to senior fitness needs. This guide is your blueprint for building a practical, budget-friendly home gym that supports your fitness journey.

Creating an Effective Home Gym on a Budget

Building a home gym doesn't require a hefty investment. With some creativity and smart shopping, you can set up an effective workout space that meets your fitness needs without breaking the bank. Here are five hints to guide you in assembling affordable gym equipment and five places where you can find these items at a budget-friendly price.

5 Hints for Affordable Gym Setup:

I. **Start with the Essentials:** Identify the types of workouts you enjoy and the equipment needed. Typically, a set of adjustable dumbbells, a yoga mat, and resistance bands can cover a wide range of exercises.

II. **Use Household Items:** Look around your home for items that can double as workout equipment. Heavy books can substitute for weights, and a sturdy chair can be used for step-ups and tricep dips.

III. **DIY Projects:** Create your own weights by filling water bottles with sand or rocks for adjustable hand weights. Similarly, a thick rope can serve as a makeshift battle rope.

IV. **Opt for Multipurpose Equipment:** Invest in items that can be used for various exercises. For example, a stability ball can be used for core workouts, weight training, and even as a bench.

V. **Go Second-Hand:** Buying used equipment can save you a significant amount, especially for higher-priced items like treadmills or stationary bikes.

5 Places to Find Affordable Gym Equipment:

I. **Online Marketplaces:** Websites like Craigslist, eBay, and Facebook Marketplace are excellent sources for finding second-hand exercise equipment at lower prices.

II.   **Garage Sales:** Keep an eye out for local garage sales. Many people sell barely-used fitness equipment for a fraction of the original price.

III.   **Thrift Stores:** Thrift stores and charity shops sometimes have exercise equipment. It's hit or miss, but you might find some hidden gems.

IV.   **Discount Retailers**: Stores like Walmart, Target, and even Aldi occasionally offer new fitness equipment at very competitive prices, especially during sales.

V.   **Fitness Forums and Community Boards:** Online communities dedicated to fitness often have sections where members sell or give away equipment they no longer use.

Creating a home gym on a budget requires patience and creativity, but it's entirely feasible. By focusing on essential equipment, considering second-hand items, and being resourceful with household objects, you can build a functional and affordable home workout space. This approach not only saves money but also supports a sustainable lifestyle by reusing and repurposing items.

Outdoor Exercises for Fresh Air and Vitamin D

Outdoor Exercises for Fresh Air and Vitamin D

Exercising outdoors not only provides the body with essential Vitamin D but also elevates mood and improves mental well-being. Here are 10 detailed outdoor exercises and activities that seniors can enjoy for health benefits and a boost in Vitamin D intake, each offering a blend of enjoyment and physical activity.

I. **Brisk Walking in a Park:**

❖ Find a local park with walking trails. Start with a 10-minute gentle walk to warm up, gradually increase your pace to a brisk walk that raises your heart rate but allows you to speak comfortably. Aim for a total of 30 minutes, followed by a cool-down walk.

II. **Gardening for Flexibility and Strength:**

❖ Engage in gardening activities such as planting, weeding, and digging. Use gardening as an opportunity to squat, stretch, and bend, promoting flexibility and muscle strength. Spend 20-30 minutes performing various gardening tasks, taking breaks as needed.

Tai Chi in the Open Air:

❖ Practice Tai Chi in your backyard or a quiet, grassy area in a park. Perform a series of Tai Chi movements focusing on fluid motions and deep breathing for 30 minutes. This promotes balance, flexibility, and stress reduction.

III. **Outdoor Yoga:**

❖ Bring a yoga mat to a peaceful outdoor location. Perform a sequence of yoga poses that focus on balance, strength, and flexibility. Include sun salutations, warrior poses, and seated stretches, holding each pose for several breaths. Practice for 30-45 minutes.

IV. **Bench Step-Ups:**

❖ Find a sturdy park bench. Step up onto the bench with one foot, bringing the other to meet it, then step down.

Alternate legs. Perform 2 sets of 10-15 step-ups per leg. This exercise strengthens the legs and improves balance.

V.   Park Bench Push-Ups:

❖ Facing a park bench, place your hands on the seat, arms shoulder-width apart. Step your feet back to form a plank position. Lower your chest towards the bench, then push up. Perform 2 sets of 10-15 push-ups, adjusting the difficulty by altering hand placement.

VI.   Light Jogging or Power Walking:

❖ On a flat, safe path, engage in light jogging or power walking. Incorporate intervals by alternating between 1 minute of jogging/power walking and 2 minutes of brisk walking. Continue for 20-30 minutes.

VII.   Cycling on Level Paths:

❖ Use a bicycle to explore park trails or a quiet neighborhood. Keep a moderate pace that allows you to feel the exertion without overdoing it. Cycle for 30-60 minutes, depending on your comfort and fitness level.

VIII.   Resistance Band Exercises:

❖ Bring a resistance band to the park. Wrap the band around a tree or a park bench for stability. Perform exercises like chest presses, rows, and leg presses. Complete 2 sets of 10-15 repetitions per exercise.

IX.   Outdoor Swimming:

❖ If you have access to a community outdoor pool, engage in swimming laps or water aerobics. The buoyancy of water makes swimming an excellent low-impact exercise for seniors, strengthening muscles and improving cardiovascular health. Swim for 20-30 minutes, adjusting the intensity as needed.

Each of these activities combines the benefits of physical exercise with the therapeutic effects of being outdoors, making them ideal for seniors seeking to improve their health and well-being. Always remember to wear sunscreen, stay hydrated, and dress appropriately for the weather to maximize the benefits of your outdoor exercise sessions.

Pool Workouts for Joint-Friendly Fitness

Water workouts are a boon for seniors, offering a joint-friendly exercise option that doesn't skimp on efficiency. This section dives into the benefits of aquatic exercise, including how water resistance and buoyancy create an ideal environment for strengthening muscles, improving endurance, and enhancing flexibility. Sample water routines are provided, focusing on exercises that are both effective and safe for seniors. Safety in and around the pool is paramount; we share advice on precautions to take, ensuring a secure and enjoyable aquatic exercise experience. Discover community resources for water aerobics classes and swim clubs that cater to seniors, making pool workouts a social and healthful part of your routine.

Pool Workouts for Joint-Friendly Fitness Exercises

Pool workouts offer a fantastic way for seniors to exercise without putting stress on their joints, thanks to the buoyancy of water. Here are 10 detailed aquatic exercises that enhance strength, flexibility, and cardiovascular health, making them perfect for seniors seeking low-impact options.

❑ **Water Walking or Jogging:**

❖ Begin in the shallow end where your feet can touch the ground. Walk from one side of the pool to the other, or jog in place if space is limited. The water resistance will increase the effort required compared to land walking. Aim for 10-15 minutes, gradually increasing the duration as your stamina improves.

❑ **Aqua Aerobics Leg Lifts:**

❖ Stand in waist-high water and hold onto the pool edge or a noodle for balance. Lift one leg to the side, then lower it back down, fighting against the water's resistance. Perform 10-15 lifts per leg, focusing on keeping your core engaged.

❑ **Pool Planks:**

❖ Use a pool noodle for this exercise. Hold the noodle in both hands, then lean forward into a plank position with the noodle under your chest. Keep your body straight and hold the position for 30 seconds to 1 minute. The water adds instability, engaging your core muscles.

❑ **Flutter Kicks:**

❖ Hold onto the pool edge or a kickboard with your arms extended. Extend your legs behind you and perform small, rapid flutter kicks. Continue for 30 seconds to 1 minute, focusing on engaging your glutes and hamstrings.

❑ Water Squats:

❖ Stand with your feet shoulder-width apart in chest-high water. Perform squats by bending at the knees and lowering your body, then pushing back up to standing. The water will help support your weight, making this easier on the knees. Complete 2 sets of 10-15 squats.

❑ Arm Curls:

❖ Use water weights or your natural resistance in the water. With palms facing up, bend your elbows to curl your arms towards your shoulders, then lower them back down. Perform 2 sets of 10-15 curls, ensuring you're moving slowly to maximize resistance.

❑ Standing Leg Extensions:

❖ Hold onto the side of the pool for support. Extend one leg out in front of you, then pull it back in. Switch legs after 10-15 extensions. Focus on keeping your movements controlled to leverage the water's resistance.

❑ Aquatic Push-Ups:

❖ Stand facing the pool wall with your hands on the edge, slightly wider than shoulder-width apart. Lean in towards the wall, then push yourself back to the starting position, as if performing a standing push-up. Complete 2 sets of 10-15 repetitions.

- **Back Wall Glide:**

  - ❖ Use the pool wall for support, placing your hands on the edge. Push off with your feet and try to glide backward as far as you can with your back straight and legs together. Pull yourself back to the starting position and repeat 10-15 times.

- **Torso Twists:**

  - ❖ Stand in waist-high water with feet planted and knees slightly bent. Extend your arms in front of you and twist your torso to one side, then to the other, allowing your hips to follow the movement slightly. Perform 2 sets of 10-15 twists to each side, engaging your core muscles.

These pool workouts provide a comprehensive routine that strengthens muscles, enhances cardiovascular fitness, and improves flexibility while minimizing the risk of joint strain. Always ensure safety by wearing water shoes for better traction and staying hydrated even while in the water.

Travel-Friendly Workouts for Seniors on the Go

Traveling doesn't mean leaving your fitness routine behind. This chapter offers strategies for staying active while exploring new places, from incorporating walks into your sightseeing plans to utilizing hotel room space for exercise. We recommend portable fitness equipment that's easy to pack and use on the go, ensuring you can maintain your workout regimen anywhere. Engage with local cultures through physical activities or sports, turning travel experiences into unique exercise opportunities. Learn how to adapt workouts to different travel scenarios, keeping your fitness on track whether you're in the air, on the road, or adjusting to new altitudes.

Travel-Friendly Workouts for Seniors on the Go Exercises

Staying active while traveling is crucial for seniors to maintain their fitness routine and overall health. Here are 10 travel-friendly workouts designed to be easily performed in a hotel room, at a park, or even in a small space, ensuring seniors can continue to exercise no matter where they are.

- **Chair Squats:**

  - ❖ Stand in front of a sturdy chair with feet hip-width apart.

  - ❖ Lower your body as if you are about to sit, then stop just above the chair and stand back up.

  - ❖ Perform 2 sets of 10-12 repetitions to strengthen your thighs and glutes.

- **Walking Lunges:**

  - ❖ In a spacious area, take a step forward with one leg and lower your hips to drop your back knee toward the floor.

  - ❖ Keep your front knee above your front ankle as you lower down.

  - ❖ Push back up and step forward, switching legs. Continue for 10 lunges on each leg.

☐ **Wall Push-Ups:**

❖ Stand arm's length away from a wall with feet shoulder-width apart.

❖ Place your hands on the wall at shoulder height and perform a push-up, bending your elbows to lower your chest to the wall, then push back.

❖ Do 2 sets of 10-12 repetitions to work your chest and arms.

☐ **Seated Leg Lifts:**

❖ Sit on the edge of a chair and extend one leg out straight.

❖ Lift the leg to hip level, then lower it back down, keeping the movements controlled.

❖ Perform 10-15 lifts on each leg to strengthen the quadriceps.

☐ **Resistance Band Pull-Aparts:**

❖ Hold a resistance band with both hands in front of you at chest height, hands wider than shoulder-width apart.

❖ Pull the band apart by moving your hands to the sides, squeezing your shoulder blades together.

❖ Slowly return to the starting position. Complete 2 sets of 12-15 repetitions.

☐ **Step-Ups:**

❖ Using a sturdy step or low bench, step up with one foot and bring the other to meet it at the top, then step back down.

❖ Alternate legs and perform 2 sets of 10-12 repetitions per leg to improve balance and leg strength.

☐ **Calf Raises:**

❖ Stand near a wall for balance and place your feet hip-width apart.

❖ Raise your heels as high as possible, then lower them back down.

❖ Perform 2 sets of 15-20 repetitions to strengthen the calf muscles.

☐ **Side Leg Raises:**

❖ Lie on your side on a yoga mat or soft surface, supporting your head with your hand.

❖ Lift your top leg toward the ceiling, then lower it back down without letting it touch the bottom leg.

❖ Do 10-15 repetitions on each side to target the outer thighs and hips.

☐ **Arm Circles:**

❖ Stand with feet shoulder-width apart and extend your arms out to the sides at shoulder Height.

❖ Make small circles with your arms, gradually increasing the size of the circles.

❖ Continue for 30 seconds, then reverse the direction for another 30 seconds to work the shoulders.

☐ **Abdominal Bracing:**

* ❖ Lie on your back with knees bent and feet flat on the floor.

* ❖ Tighten your abdominal muscles as if bracing for impact, holding for 5-10 seconds.

* ❖ Relax and repeat. Perform 2 sets of 10-15 repetitions to strengthen the core muscles.

These exercises offer a versatile workout that can be adapted to any travel situation, helping seniors stay fit and active on the go. They require minimal equipment and space, making them ideal for maintaining a workout routine while traveling.

Incorporating Movement into Daily Chores

Turn daily chores into a fitness routine with functional fitness principles. This section provides creative ways to enhance physical activity through everyday tasks like gardening, cleaning, and shopping. Transform these chores into opportunities to practice balance, coordination, and strength in a practical, functional context. We also emphasize ergonomic practices, ensuring that daily activities promote health rather than contribute to strain or injury. By integrating movement into your chores, you not only accomplish your tasks but also contribute to your overall fitness goals, making every action an opportunity for improvement.

Incorporating Movement into Daily Chores Exercises

Integrating exercise into daily chores can transform routine tasks into opportunities for physical activity, making fitness a natural part of your day. Here are 10 examples of how seniors can incorporate movement and workouts into their daily chores, turning mundane activities into beneficial exercises.

☐ **Vacuum Lunges:**

❖ While vacuuming, step forward into a lunge with each push of the vacuum. Alternate legs to work both sides evenly. This helps strengthen the legs and improve balance.

☐ **Calf Raises While Washing Dishes:**

❖ Stand at the sink and perform calf raises by lifting your heels off the ground and then lowering them. This can be done while washing dishes or preparing food. Aim for 3 sets of 15 repetitions.

☐ **Countertop Push-Ups:**

❖ While waiting for the kettle to boil or during a cooking downtime, use the kitchen counter to perform push-ups. Place your hands on the edge of the counter, step back so your body at an angle, and perform push-ups to strengthen your arms and chest.

☐ **Laundry Squats:**

❖ Each time you load or unload the laundry machine, perform a squat. Make sure to keep your back straight and bend at the knees. This is a great way to work on leg strength and flexibility.

❑ **Stair Step-Ups:**

❖ If you have stairs at home, make extra trips up and down or simply step up and down on the bottom step multiple times for a cardio and leg strengthening workout.

❑ **Gardening Lunges:**

❖ When gardening, use lunges to reach for weeds or plants instead of bending over from the waist. This can help maintain leg strength and improve flexibility.

❑ **Towel Grip Strengthens:**

❖ While holding a towel (either after laundry or during folding), grip it tightly and release. Repeat this several times to improve hand and forearm strength.

❑ **Grocery Bag Curls:**

❖ Use grocery bags as weights for bicep curls. Ensure the bags are evenly weighted and perform curls as you carry them to the kitchen. Aim for 2 sets of 10 curls with each arm.

❑ **Balance on One Foot While Brushing Teeth:**

❖ Stand on one foot while brushing your teeth to improve balance and core strength. Switch feet halfway through. Lean against the sink or wall if you need extra support.

D Dancing While Dusting:

❖ Put on your favorite music and dance around the house while dusting or wiping surfaces. Dancing improves cardiovascular health and flexibility, and it makes chores more enjoyable.

Incorporating these movements into your daily chores not only helps in maintaining physical activity but also breaks the monotony, making everyday tasks more engaging and beneficial for your health. Always listen to your body and modify activities to suit your fitness level and abilities.

Sources:

https://www.verywellfit.com/best-exercise-equipment-for-seniors-7563564

https://www.ncbi.nlm.nih.gov/pmc/articles/PMC3546779/

https://www.ncbi.nlm.nih.gov/pmc/articles/PMC3820233/

https://www.silversneakers.com/blog/travel-workout/

Chapter 7

Overcoming Common Obstacles

<u>Busting the "Too Old to Exercise" Myth</u>

The belief that age is a barrier to fitness is a myth that this chapter aims to dismantle. We confront ageist stereotypes head-on, showcasing inspiring stories of seniors who have embarked on their fitness journeys later in life, proving it's never too late to start. Fitness is not one-size-fits-all; it's highly adaptable to individual health and mobility levels, offering something for everyone, regardless of age. This section highlights the unique advantages that come with age, such as patience, wisdom, and a refined sense of self-awareness, which can enhance the exercise experience. Additionally, we provide a wealth of resources designed to support seniors new to exercise, ensuring that beginning a fitness routine is accessible and rewarding.

Busting the "Too Old to Exercise" Myth Daily Affirmations

The belief that one can be "too old to exercise" is a myth that needs to be dispelled. Exercise is beneficial at any age, especially for seniors, as it can improve physical health, enhance mental well-being, and increase quality of life. Here are three motivational daily affirmations designed to inspire seniors to embrace physical activity regardless of age:

D "Every Movement Counts Towards My Health and Vitality."

❖ This affirmation encourages the recognition that all forms of movement, no matter how small, contribute positively to overall health. It emphasizes that there's no minimum threshold for exercise to be beneficial, promoting a more inclusive and achievable approach to fitness for seniors.

D "I Am Capable of Improving My Strength and Balance Today."

❖ Focusing on the present, this affirmation motivates seniors to take actionable steps towards enhancing their physical capabilities. It reinforces the idea that strength and balance can always be improved, fostering a growth mindset that challenges the misconception that aging inherently limits physical improvement.

D "Age is Just a Number; My Will to Stay Active Defines Me."

❖ This powerful statement serves as a reminder that age should not dictate one's ability to engage in physical activity. It highlights personal determination as the defining factor in maintaining an active lifestyle, encouraging seniors to redefine societal expectations about aging and exercise.

By integrating these affirmations into daily routines, seniors can shift their mindset from viewing age as a barrier to seeing it as an opportunity for continued growth and well-being through exercise.

Solutions for When You're Short on Time

Time constraints are a common hurdle, but they shouldn't keep you from maintaining an active lifestyle. This chapter introduces the concept of micro-workouts—short, yet effective, exercise sessions that can easily fit into a busy schedule. We explore practical ways to integrate more physical activity into daily life, such as utilizing standing desks or opting for walking meetings. Tips for prioritizing and planning ensure that exercise becomes a non-negotiable part of your routine, emphasizing the selection of efficient exercises that maximize benefits within limited time frames.

Solutions for When You're Short on Time Workouts and Solutions

Finding time for exercise can be challenging, especially with a busy schedule. However, incorporating physical activity into your day doesn't always require long sessions at the gym. Here are three quick and easy solutions for fitting workout time into a typical day, ensuring you stay active even when you're short on time.

I.   **Micro-Workouts Throughout the Day:**

   ❖ Break down your exercise routine into short, manageable sessions that can be spread throughout the day. For example, commit to 5 minutes of physical activity every hour. This could be a set of squats, wall push-ups, or stretching. These micro-workouts can add up to a substantial amount of exercise by the end of the day and can be easily integrated into breaks at work or moments at home.

II. **Incorporate Physical Activity into Daily Tasks:**

   ❖ Turn routine activities into opportunities for exercise. Walk or bike to the store instead of driving, take the stairs instead of the elevator, or do calf raises while standing in line.

These small changes can increase your physical activity without requiring extra time out of your day.

III.   High-Intensity Interval Training (HIIT) Workouts:

- ❖ HIIT workouts are designed to deliver maximum benefits in minimal time by alternating short bursts of intense exercise with brief periods of rest or lower-intensity exercise. A full HIIT session can be completed in as little as 10 to 20 minutes. You can find numerous HIIT routines online that require no equipment and can be performed in a small space. This makes HIIT an ideal solution for a quick workout that effectively boosts your heart rate and burns calories.

By adopting these strategies, you can ensure that time constraints do not hinder your fitness goals. Integrating physical activity into your daily routine, even in short bursts, can significantly contribute to your overall health and well-being.

Adapting Workouts for Limited Mobility

Limited mobility does not equate to limited options when it comes to exercise. This section is dedicated to customizing workout plans that accommodate mobility challenges, ensuring every individual can safely and effectively participate in physical activity. The importance of professional guidance is underscored, highlighting how physical therapists and specialized fitness professionals can tailor exercises to meet specific needs. We also discuss the role of accessibility tools and technology in facilitating exercise, and the benefits of joining inclusive fitness communities that offer support and adaptation tips for those with mobility concerns.

Adapting Workouts for Limited Mobility WheelChair Bound Exercises

For individuals who are wheelchair-bound, staying active is crucial for health and well-being. Here are five safe workout activities specifically designed to accommodate limited mobility, focusing on enhancing strength, flexibility, and cardiovascular health without the need for standing or walking.

- **Wheelchair Push-ups:**

  - ❖ Sit in your wheelchair or a sturdy chair without wheels, if possible. Place your hands on the armrests.

  - ❖ Push down on the armrests to lift your body slightly off the seat, then slowly lower yourself back down.

  - ❖ This exercise strengthens the arms, shoulders, and chest. Aim for 2 sets of 8-10 repetitions.

- **Seated Resistance Band Rows:**

  - ❖ Secure a resistance band around a stable, immovable object at waist level when seated.

  - ❖ Hold the ends of the band with both hands, arms extended, then pull the band towards your waist, squeezing your shoulder blades together.

  - ❖ Slowly return to the starting position. Perform 2 sets of 10-12 repetitions to strengthen tieback and improve posture.

- **Upper Body Circles:**

  - ❖ Extend your arms straight out to the sides at shoulder height.

- ❖ Slowly make small circles with your arms, gradually increasing the size of the circles.

- ❖ After 30 seconds, reverse the direction of the circles. This activity enhances shoulder flexibility and can help alleviate upper body tension.

☐ **Seated Torso Twists:**

- ❖ Sit upright with your feet flat on the ground (if your feet don't reach the ground, they can hang or rest on footrests).

- ❖ Place your hands on your shoulders or cross your arms over your chest.

- ❖ Gently twist your torso to the right as far as is comfortable, return to center, then twist to the Left.

- ❖ Perform 2 sets of 10-12 twists on each side to improve core strength and spinal flexibility.

☐ **Seated Leg Lifts:**

- ❖ If you have some mobility in your legs, try seated leg lifts to strengthen the thigh muscles.

- ❖ Sit upright and extend one leg out straight, then lift it as high as possible. Slowly lower it back down.

- ❖ If you're unable to lift the leg completely, even a partial lift or attempting the motion can be beneficial.

- ❖ Perform 10 lifts per leg, aiming for 2 sets.

These exercises are designed to be performed safely within the constraints of limited mobility, allowing those who are wheelchair-bound to engage in physical activity. Always consult with a healthcare provider before beginning any new exercise regimen, particularly to ensure that the activities are appropriate for your specific health condition and mobility level.

Keeping Exercise Interesting to Avoid Boredom

Variety is the spice of life, and this is especially true when it comes to exercise. To combat boredom and sustain interest in physical activity, this chapter encourages diversifying your workout routine. Trying new sports, joining different fitness classes, or exploring novel activities can rekindle enthusiasm for exercise. Setting personal challenges or participating in community fitness challenges provides motivation and a sense of accomplishment. Implementing a rewards system for reaching exercise milestones can further enhance engagement, making the pursuit of fitness a continually rewarding and enjoyable experience.

Keeping Exercise Interesting to Avoid Boredom Tips and Tricks

Maintaining an exercise routine can sometimes become monotonous, leading to a lack of motivation. To keep your workouts engaging and productive, here are five hints or tricks to avoid boredom and sustain interest in your fitness journey.

I.   **Mix Up Your Routine:**

- ❖ Change your workout plan every few weeks by incorporating different types of exercises or activities. This not only prevents boredom but also challenges different muscle groups and improves overall fitness. For example, if you usually go for walks, try adding cycling or swimming into your routine. Variety keeps both the mind and body engaged.

II.   **Set New Goals:**

- ❖ Continuously setting new, achievable goals keeps motivation high and gives you something to work towards. Whether it's improving your time, increasing your reps, or mastering a new exercise, having clear objectives can reinvigorate your workout routine. Celebrate when you reach these milestones to acknowledge your progress.

III.   **Workout with Friends or Join a Group:**

- ❖ Exercising with friends or joining a fitness class can introduce a social aspect to your workouts, making them more enjoyable and less like a chore. The camaraderie and gentle competition can motivate you to push harder and make the time fly by. Plus, you're less likely to skip a workout when others are counting on your presence.

IV.   **Incorporate Technology:**

- ❖ Use fitness apps or online platforms to discover new workouts, track your progress, and stay engaged. Many apps offer challenges, virtual rewards, and community support to keep you motivated. Additionally, streaming services provide countless fitness classes that can bring fresh and exciting workouts right into your living room.

V.   **Connect Exercise to Your Interests:**

- ❖ Tailor your exercise routine to include activities you genuinely enjoy. If you love nature, opt for hikes or outdoor yoga. If music energizes you, create a dynamic playlist for your workouts or engage in dance fitness. When exercise aligns with your interests, it feels less like a duty and more like a fun part of your day.

By implementing these strategies, you can transform your exercise routine into a dynamic and enjoyable aspect of your lifestyle,

keeping boredom at bay and ensuring long-term commitment to
your fitness goals.

<u>Staying Hydrated: Tips and Tricks</u>

Staying Hydrated: Tips and Tricks

For seniors, maintaining hydration is essential during workouts to
ensure optimal performance and overall health. Here are five tips
and tricks for staying hydrated, along with five ideal drinks that
can help seniors stay hydrated during their fitness routines.

5 Tips and Tricks for Staying Hydrated:

- **Start Hydrated:**

  - Begin your exercise routine already well-hydrated. Drink
    water consistently in the hours leading up to your workout,
    not just right before you start.

- **Schedule Drink Breaks:**

  - Set a timer or plan specific times in your workout to take
    breaks for drinking water. This is especially important as
    seniors may have a reduced sensation of thirst.

- **Monitor Your Hydration:**

  - Pay attention to signs of dehydration, which can include
    dry mouth, fatigue, and dark-colored urine. Use these signs
    as indicators that you need to increase your fluid intake.

❑ **Use a Reusable Water Bottle:**

❖ Keep a reusable water bottle within reach during your workout. Choosing one with measurement markings can help you track how much you're drinking.

❑ **Hydrate Throughout the Day:**

❖ Don't limit hydration to workout times only. Drink fluids consistently throughout the day to maintain hydration levels, especially before and after exercising.

5 Ideal Drinks for Hydration:

Water:

❖ The best, most straightforward choice for staying hydrated. It's calorie-free, cost-effective, and readily available.

Coconut Water:

❖ A natural source of electrolytes, particularly potassium, making it a great option for rehydration post-workout. Choose the unsweetened varieties to avoid extra sugar.

Electrolyte-Infused Water:

❖ These are especially formulated waters that contain added electrolytes (like sodium and potassium) without the added sugars and calories of traditional sports drinks, making them a good option for maintaining electrolyte balance.

Herbal Tea (Chilled or Lukewarm):

❖ Non-caffeinated herbal teas can be a flavorful way to increase your water intake. Drinking them chilled or lukewarm can provide variety without the diuretic effects of caffeine.

Diluted Fruit Juice:

❖ Diluting natural fruit juice with water or sparkling water reduces the sugar content while still providing flavor and some electrolytes. This can be a refreshing option, particularly after exercising.

Staying hydrated is key to a successful fitness routine, especially for seniors. By implementing these hydration tips and incorporating these drinks into your regimen, you can help ensure that your body remains well-hydrated, supporting your overall health and workout performance.

Sources:

https://www.americansportandfitness.com/blogs/fitness-blog/success-stories-from-senior-fitness-training

https://www.healthline.com/health/everyday-fitness/senior-workouts

https://seniorfitness4life.com/how-to-stay-fit-as-a-senior-find-an-exercise-buddy/

Conclusion

As we bring our journey through "Top 50+ Workouts for Seniors" to a close, let's revisit the empowering truth that it's never too late to embark on a fitness journey. This book has been a testament to the transformative power of exercise, tailored to meet the unique needs of seniors. With a focus on low-impact, balance, and strength training exercises, we've laid out a path to enhance daily living, ensuring that each workout is not just an activity to lose weight, but a step toward a healthier, more vibrant life.

Our core message has been clear: senior fitness is about adopting a holistic approach that encompasses not only physical exercises but also nutrition, hydration, and the mind-body connection. This comprehensive strategy underscores the role of proper nutrition and mental well-being in achieving overall health and fitness.

The adaptable and customizable nature of the workouts presented in this book ensures that everyone, regardless of their starting point, can find a routine that resonates with them. We've encouraged you to weave fitness into the fabric of your daily life, transforming it from a chore into a source of joy and a significant enhancer of your quality of life.

Now, the ball is in your court. The first step might seem daunting, but remember, the journey of a thousand miles begins with a single step. Set realistic goals, track your progress, and don't forget to celebrate every achievement along the way. Embrace the support of a community, whether it's through senior-specific fitness classes, community groups, or online forums, to keep the motivation burning and the workouts enjoyable.

Yes, there will be challenges, and there might be days when your motivation dips. However, with persistence, adaptability, and a focus on the myriad benefits awaiting you, pushing through becomes not just possible, but inevitable. Envision the active, fulfilled life that lies ahead: more independence, the joy of engaging in hobbies and activities you love, improved health, and the sheer pleasure of living life to its fullest.

As Pilar Patel, I leave you with a part of my heart in these pages. Fitness has been a transformative force in my life, and my deepest hope is that this book serves as both a guide and inspiration for you to discover the joy and myriad benefits of a healthier, more active lifestyle.

Your journey doesn't end here; it evolves. I invite you to share your stories, progress, and insights. Reach out via email or visit our website to join a community of like-minded individuals embarking on this rewarding path. Together, let's celebrate every step, every stretch, and every stride towards a healthier tomorrow.

With warmth and encouragement,

Pilar Patel

Epilogue
Make a Difference with Your Review!
Unlock the Power of Generosity

People who give without expecting anything in return often live longer, happier lives and are more successful. So, let's try to make a difference together!

Our mission is to make workouts for seniors accessible to everyone, especially seniors over 60. Everything I do stems from that mission. And the only way for us to accomplish that mission is by reaching…
well…everyone.

Please help that senior by leaving this book a review. Your gift costs no money and takes less than 60 seconds, but it can change a fellow senior's life forever. Your review could help…

…one more senior to reclaim balance.

…one more person to lose weight.

…one more individual feels happier and healthier.

To get that 'feel good' feeling and help this person for real, all you have to do is…and it takes less than 60 seconds…

Leave a review.

https://amzn.to/3YQGbQO

Please Leave a review.